YOUR KNOWLEDGE HAS VALUE

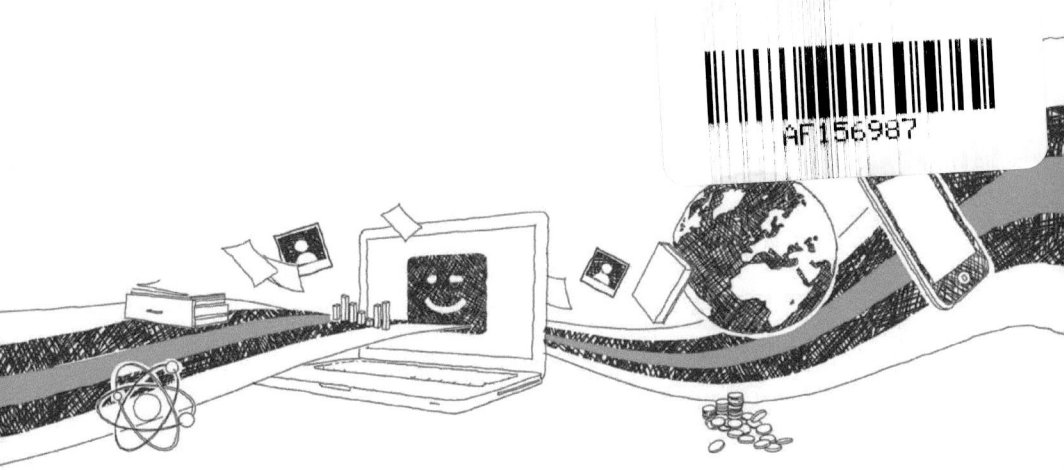

- We will publish your bachelor's and master's thesis, essays and papers

- Your own eBook and book - sold worldwide in all relevant shops

- Earn money with each sale

Upload your text at www.GRIN.com and publish for free

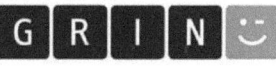

Bibliographic information published by the German National Library:

The German National Library lists this publication in the National Bibliography; detailed bibliographic data are available on the Internet at http://dnb.dnb.de .

Imprint:

Copyright © 2017 GRIN Verlag, Open Publishing GmbH
Print and binding: Books on Demand GmbH, Norderstedt Germany
ISBN: 9783668596795

This book at GRIN:

https://www.grin.com/document/383683

Hyder Mirghani

The interaction of type 2 diabetes, type 3 diabetes (Alzheimer's disease), and the gut microbiota

GRIN Publishing

GRIN - Your knowledge has value

Since its foundation in 1998, GRIN has specialized in publishing academic texts by students, college teachers and other academics as e-book and printed book. The website www.grin.com is an ideal platform for presenting term papers, final papers, scientific essays, dissertations and specialist books.

Visit us on the internet:

http://www.grin.com/

http://www.facebook.com/grincom

http://www.twitter.com/grin_com

The interaction of type 2 diabetes, type 3 diabetes (Alzheimer's disease), and the gut microbiota

Hyder Osman Mirghani MD, MSc, DCN, Assistant Professor of Medicine, and Endocrine, Medical College, University of Tabuk, Saudi Arabia

Contents

Chapter 1. Introduction

Dementia is a multifaceted syndrome with a significant public health, social, and economic burden; there are forty-four million people affected by the disease worldwide according to the most recent estimate. The number is projected to double by the year 2030 and to triple by 2050 (1,2).

Alzheimer's disease (AD, or type-3 diabetes mellitus) and vascular dementia are the most common forms of dementia. Lifestyle risk factors including obesity and type 2 diabetes increase the risk for the development of both vascular and nonvascular dementia in later life. Previous literature reported that people with diabetes mellitus had 70% greater risk for dementia development (3). Traditionally, type-2 diabetes and AD (type-3 diabetes) have been thought as independent disorders; recent literature suggests possible links that could lead to common effective modalities of treatment. Furthermore, the highly innervated pancreas shares many features with the brain at molecular levels (4).

Metformin is recommended as the first line for the treatment of patients with type 2 diabetes mellitus due to its effectiveness, favorable effects on lipids and cardiovascular risks, and safety profile. The previous restriction of the use of metformin in patients with the moderate renal disease is loosened by the Food and Drug Organization(5,6). Thus the use of this valuable and affordable drug is expected to increase.

The American Diabetes Association recommended the periodic measurement of vitamin B12 and supplementation as needed to reflect the recent evidence showing the association of long-term use of metformin and B12 deficiency (6). Although the role of vitamin B12 deficiency in the development of dementia is well-established, the role of metformin in B12 deficiency and dementia remain to be elucidated (7,8).

Insulin resistance is considered as a primary factor for the association of diabetes mellitus and dementia. However, the role of insulin sensitizer in the prevention of dementia remains unclear(9). Furthermore, there is an increasing concern about the role of metformin in cognitive disorders (10). Thus we conducted this narrative review, in this study we reviewed the literature to assess the interaction of Alzheimer's disease, the gut, and its microbiome, and to assess the role of metformin and other drugs used for type 1&2 diabetes mellitus as possible therapies for the AD. The role of microbiota and fecal transplantation on cognitive disorders was also discussed.

Chapter 2.Prevalence &Pathogenesis of type 3 diabetes mellitus

Dementia is characterized by global progressive cognitive dysfunction including learning, memory, speech, comprehension, orientation, and judgment. The most common form of dementia is Alzheimer's disease (AD) accounting for more than 60%. Due to the increasing aging population, the disease is on the rise. Currently, 36 million people were affected worldwide and the projection for the year 2050 is > 115 million. Dementia poses a significant burden on the patients, family, healthcare system, and the community as a whole (11-13).

Glucose is an essential energy source for human body function. The regulation of this vital energy involves the interaction of the liver, the pancreas, and brain. Glucose is converted to lactate by astrocytes; this lactate is essential for neuronal metabolism, the expression of genes involved in memory, and the formation of dendrites and synapses. The disruption of the physiological balance could result in metabolic compromise leading to diabetes including type-3 diabetes (AD). Age is an essential risk factor for both type-2 and type-3 diabetes mellitus, as the brain ages it becomes more liable to cell damage induced with high plasma sugar and this could explain the development of cognitive impairment observed in some patients with diabetes. The brain is highly susceptible to plasma glucose perpetuation, and both hypoglycemia and hyperglycemia are dangerous (14).

Alzheimer's disease (AD) a degenerative brain disease is also called type 3 diabetes. It is the most frequent cause of dementia and characterized by extracellular amyloid beta (Aβ) plaques and intraneuronal deposits of neurofibrillary tangles (NFTs). Due to the increasing age of the population, the disease is on the rise worldwide. The growing rate of AD among older adults is also associated with the uprise in obesity and type 2 diabetes mellitus. Thus many consider AD as a metabolic disease. The diseases share many features including risk factors, demographic profiles, and clinical and biochemical characteristics. Antioxidant, insulin and adiponectin were suggested as mechanisms linking the three disorders. Previous literature reported reduced insulin signal transductions in the brain. Furthermore, insulin injected (intranasal) has been shown to affect AD treatment. Also, oxidative stress induction by Aβ and NFTs and the reduced levels of adiponectin observed among patients with type 2 diabetes and obesity are suggested as causes for the metabolic dysfunction in both the brain and other organs linking AD to obesity and type 2 diabetes (15).

Alzheimer's disease is often called brain diabetes or type 3 diabetes mellitus because it showed reduced neuronal insulin receptors and insulin expression with the ultimate breakdown of insulin signaling pathway (the bases of insulin resistance). These observations led scientist to suggest that AD is a neuroendocrine disorder resembling type 2 diabetes mellitus in term of insulin resistance that leads to brain metabolic disturbances and cognitive impairment (16). Due to the shared cellular and molecular features in type 1, type 2 diabetes, and insulin resistance associated with cognitive decline and memory loss among the elderly population, the researchers proposed the term type 3 diabetes for Alzheimer's disease. The AD has composite features of insulin deficiency and insulin resistance (both type-1 and type 2 diabetes mellitus). Insulin is involved in the activation of glycogen synthase kinase 3β, to phosphorylate tau, the latter is involved in the formation of neurofibrillary tangles. Interestingly, insulin also plays a principal role in amyloid plaques formation (17). Another substance that can alter the mechanism involved in type 2 diabetes and Alzheimer's disease is Humanin a recently introduced, mitochondrial-derived peptide with neuroprotective effects (18).

6

Lifestyle modification could play an essential role in the prevention of AD. Previous literature showed that modifiable cardiovascular risk factors could increase the risk of the AD. Furthermore, physical inactivity and smoking constitute 37.7% of the population attributable (19). A lifestyle prevention program targeting both type 2 &3 diabetes mellitus is highly beneficial. The Mediterranean diet rich in fruits, vegetable, whole grain, moderate consumption of dairy products, polyunsaturated fatty acids, and low meat consumption has been shown to improve cognitive dysfunction. Mediterranean diet as a dietary pattern, the individual nutrients characteristic of this food, and other micronutrients like vitamins (C, E, and B-12) and flavonoids reduce oxidative stress and low grade inflammation and positively affect cognitive dysfunction (20). It is interesting to note that, the relationship between type-2 diabetes and type-3 diabetes is bidirectional. Patients with the AD are more susceptible to type-2 diabetes mellitus, AD-implicated brain dysfunction in the pathogenesis of T2DM could be possible. AD is also associated with chronic inflammation, oxidative stress and impaired cognition as well as metabolic alterations, including impaired neuronal insulin signaling, impaired cerebral energy metabolism, and reduced glucose metabolism. Whether these shared characteristics are due to obesity which is common in both type-3 and type-2 diabetes and if they are fixed or reversible needs further research. Obesity, type-2 diabetes and the chronic consumption of a high-fat diet (especially saturated fat)　have been linked to reduced cognitive function in both animals and human studies, with some improvement with a healthier friendly diet Furthermore, AD mouse models crossed with genetic mouse models of diabetes (such as *ob/ob* and *db/db*), show early spatial learning and memory impairments(21).

Chapter 3. Proposed Treatment for type 3 diabetes (AD)

Patients with type -2 diabetes have higher rates of dementia (50-150% increased risk). AD is the commonest form of dementia and can be due to genes or sporadic. The latter is associated with seven modifiable risk factors namely: diabetes mellitus, obesity, physical inactivity, hypertension at middle age, smoking, lower level of education, and depression. Although a framework linking the neuropathological abnormalities in Alzheimer's disease is lacking, there is accumulating evidence that links the neuro-cognitive dysfunction to insulin deficiency and resistance. Given the above and the fact that most of the treatment of AD failed in the stage-3 trial, it could be possible that antihyperglycemic medications may be useful in AD (22).

Intranasal insulin spray: Trial on this type of therapy showed improvement in cognitive function especially among APOE-ε4 positive genotype. The dose was 201U; the APOE-ε4 negative genotype showed improvement at higher doses. The intranasal approach was used due to efficient insulin delivery through the olfactory and trigeminal perivascular channels and axonal pathways and a lower hypoglycemia risk (22). The side effects intranasal insulin are irritation, increasing blood pressure, and nasal mucosal damage. Delivering insulin directly to the brain could overcome these side effects, but the blood-brain barrier needs to be defeated (4).

Thiazolidinediones: Due to the unwanted effects, there is a restriction of these drugs and black box warning in some countries. A large trial recruiting 500 patients with AD showed cognitive improvement among APOE-ε4-negative patients (23). The extracellular accumulation ofamyloid β in the brain and the subsequent robust inflammatory response triggered are controlled by nuclear receptors, including the liver X receptors (LXRs) and peroxisome-proliferator receptor γ (PPARγ).Skerrett et

8

al. in their animal study (24) observed that both LXRs andPPARγ agonists were associated with a lower deposition of amyloid β. Furthermore, the combination of the two agonists had a higher positive effect on cognitive dysfunction. A literature review (25) published in the year 2011 recommended against the use of PPARγ in the management of AD due to lack of efficacy and safety concerns. A randomized controlled trial (26) conducted among patients with mild cognitive dysfunction(not included in the previous review search) reported the improvement in cognitive dysfunction among patients taking pioglitazone, but no improvement in plasma Aβ40/Aβ42 ratio. A more recent (searched through December 2014 and published 2016) meta-analysis (27) stated that, in spite of the insufficient evidence for the current use, PPAR-γ agonists might be a promising therapeutic approach in future, especially pioglitazone, with large-scale randomized controlled trials to confirm. Another meta-analysis (28) conducted in the same period concluded similar findings. On the other hands, some studies (29) questioned the effects of PPAR-γ agonists on AD. More studies (30) stated the beneficial effects of PPAR-γ agonists in restoring cerebrovascular dysfunctions. Recent literature (31) suggested combination therapy for the treatment of AD due to the interaction of several subcellular factors affecting astrocytes, neurons, and capillaries. The available drugs are lithium, valproate, pioglitazone, erythropoietin, and prazosin. With some studies showing some success using pioglitazone (32,33), the TOMMORROW Trial (34) will incorporate 6000 cognitively normal subjects and randomize them to either pioglitazone or placebo. The translocase of outer mitochondrial membrane 40 homolog gene (TOMM40 gene) which is linked to APOE4 and has been shown to predict the age of late-onset AD will be targeted (35).

GLP-1R agonists and DPP-IV inhibitors: GLP-1R agonists are an attractive option because they activate pathways common to bypassing IRs and boost insulin-related signaling pathways through G protein-dependent signaling. GLP-1 like preceptors agonists are structurally not similar and bind to different receptors. They readily cross the blood-brain barriers and less likely to cause hypoglycemia, so no problem with dosing. Animal studies showed that Exendin-4 and liraglutide restored impaired insulin signaling, exerting neuroprotective effects on neurons and synapses, improving cognition, and decreasing Aβ accumulation in the brain. Furthermore, GLP-1 agonists increase cell proliferation and facilitate neuronal network repair (36,37). Amylin secreted by pancreatic cells has limited endogenous utility due to precipitation and plaques and oligomers formation. Abnormal Amylin has been reported in the brain of patients with AD, and sometimes localized with Aβ amyloid. Amylin receptors are widely distributed in the brain substance and can readily cross the blood-brain barrier, so it is suggested to have widespread implications for mood, memory anxiety, and satiety, Pramlintide soluble, non aggregating synthetic analog of amylin that lower plasma glucose by insulin release, glucagon inhibition, decreased gastric emptying, and reduced appetite has been shown to improve cognition, and inhibit inflammation and oxidative stress in the hippocampus and cortex in animals models (38,39). The minimal side effects, excellent safety profile, and tolerability of this drug are appealing for the study and treatment of Alzheimer's disease. A recent prospective study conducted among elderly diabetic patients with and without dementia showed that sitagliptin (a DPP-IV inhibitor) is associated improved cognitive dysfunction in both study groups (40). A multi-center observational study (41) conducted in Japan investigated various diabetes medications use among patients with diabetes and dementia. The study assessed the family support, ease of use, resources, and an obstacle to insulin and other medications. The authors concluded that   DPP-IV inhibitors were the appropriate drugs for patients suffering from both diabetes mellitus and dementia.

Insulin secretagogues (Glimiperide and glipizide):

In addition to pancreas stimulation, Glimiperide has extra-pancreatic functions through which it suppresses amyloid beta (Aβ) plaques and neurofibrillary tangles leading to improvement in cognitive abilities :

- ✓ Increase glucose uptake
- ✓ PPARγ activation
- ✓ Activation of GPI-anchored proteins
- ✓ suppression of BACE1 activity

The above actions indicated the promising effect of Glimiperide in the treatment of AD associated with type-2 diabetes mellitus (42-44)

Other proposed treatments:

Insulin-degrading enzyme (IDE) and Neprilysin (NEP): by degradation of Aβ plaques. The latter together with tau-neurofibrillary tangles are the basis of AD pathology, the degradation of Aβ plaques could prevent their adverse effects on insulin coding genes and insulin signaling to decrease insulin resistance, low-grade inflammation, and neurocognitive dysfunction observed in patients with Alzheimer's disease (45).

Rapamycin (mTOR): Mtor is an essential component of a complex protein which is a critical role in some signaling pathways necessary for cellular metabolic homeostasis, insulin secretion, insulin resistance pancreatic β-cell function, stem cell proliferation and differentiation, and programmed cell death with apoptosis and autophagy. Rapamycin is very promising as a future regenerative therapy for patients with type 3 and types 2 diabetes, but obstacles are on the way:

- Mtor acts through many critical pathways including, phosphoinositide 3-kinase (PI 3-K), protein kinase B (Akt), AMP-activated protein kinase (AMPK). So Mtor may not function individually, but dependent on other pathways which could limit protective paths leading to unwanted side effects like reducing the efficacy of metformin which also involve the same pathway to work. Vasculopathy is another serious side effect which needs to be addressed in future studies. Mtor plays an important role in stem cell survival; again a delicate balance is warranted in apoptotic and autophagic pathways to reach the goal of regeneration of various cell types and avoiding cell death on the other hand (46)

Centrally active angiotensin-converting enzyme inhibitors (ACE-Is): ACE inhibitors are used in various medical conditions including heart failure, kidney disease, high blood pressure, and diabetes. Evidence exists that these agents could improve cognitive function in early-stage AD through a possible anti-inflammatory effect and not merely blood pressure lowering. Thus a timely introduction of centrally active ACE-I (e.g., captopril, fosinopril, lisinopril, perindopril, ramipril, or trandolapril) could be of help in prevention and deployment of AD (47).

A page on diet side effects including organ atrophy

Chapter 4. Metformin and type 3 diabetes mellitus

Theoretically, most antihyperglycemic medication can address insulin resistance, and insulin deficiency characterized AD, but metformin is preferred due to the following:

✓ Low risk of hypoglycemia and weight loss

✓ Favorable effects on lipids and blood pressure

✓ Anticancer effects

✓ The role of metformin in Alzheimer,s disease (type 3 diabetes) is controversial. Metformin has been shown to reduce vitamin B12 levels on chronic use (The American Diabetes Association recommended to check for Vitamin B12 level and treat when appropriate) which could lead to cognitive impairment, on the other hands decreasing insulin resistance and the favorable effects on gut microbiota may enhance cognitive function.

Animal studies on metformin and AD:

Animal experiments using mouse model showed that metformin reduces tau phosphorylation in the cortex and hippocampus, increases the amount of insoluble tau and the number of inclusions with β-sheet aggregates in the brain, and exacerbates hindlimb atrophy. The study suggests that brain insulin resistance is due to Aβ pathology and is independent of peripheral insulin resistance or type 2 diabetes mellitus (48,49). The studies pointed that in spite the markers of insulin resistance are impeded in tau protein the role of tauopathology in insulin resistance is unclear and seemed to work independently (49,50). More studies showed that insulin acts in type 2 diabetes only via inhibition of mitochondrial complexes and AMPK activation independent of insulin signaling (51,52). Furthermore and surprisingly, chronic metformin use increased the amount of insoluble tau and β-sheet inclusion in the cortex and hippocampus. The studies concluded that metformin pro-aggregation effects mitigate the potential benefits arising from its dephosphorylating action. Another study conducted on C57B6/J mice found that metformin leads to an increased risk of the AD via the promotion and aggregation of β-amyloid (Aβ), in the cortex (53). Son et al. (54) conducted a study using SH-SY5Y cells and drew similar conclusions. Further reviews (55) on LAN5 neuroblastoma cells showed that metformin promotes aggregation of Aβ, induces oxidative stress, and mitochondrial damage through increments of APP and presenilin levels, proteins involved in the AD.McNeilly and colleagues (56) in their study on rats fed a high-fat diet, debated the occurrence of brain insulin resistance. The author stated that metformin affects the metabolic but not the cognitive function suggesting other pathways through which a high-fat diet affects the cognitive abilities. A more recent study (10) investigated the long-term effects of metformin on brain neurotrophins and cognition in aged male C57Bl/6 mice and concluded the following: in spite of metformin attenuation of decline motor function induced by a high-fat diet it should be approached with caution as it also decreased expression of the antioxidant pathway regulator.

Studies are showing favorable effects of metformin on cognitive functions: An experimental study (57) conducted on hippocampus cells showed that metformin mediated its protective effects through phospho-JNK but had no effect on phospho-p38 MAPK and phospho-ERK1/2. Furthermore, metformin protected against apoptosis. Chiang and colleagues (58) reported the same, but the finding of proactive role of metformin against Aβ protein aggregates was mediated at least in part through AMP-activated protein kinase (AMPK). A further study (59) using murine primary neurons from wild-type and human tau transgenic mice suggested another pathway for metformin protection against tauopathy (protein phosphatase 2A (PP2A). The investigators reported that:

- ✓ The tau dephosphorylating potency can be blocked entirely by the PP2A inhibitors okadaic acid and fostriecin, confirming that PP2A is an essential mediator of the observed effects
- ✓ Metformin effects on PP2A activity and tau phosphorylation seem to be independent of AMPK activation

A randomized controlled trial (60) conducted on male Wistar rats showed that metformin decreased the effects of Aβ on long-term potentiation in the hippocampus, so it is neuroprotective. Further animal and cell line studies (61-62) have concluded the neuroprotective effect of metformin on cognitive impairment.

Studies among humans:

A study published in the year 2009 concluded that metformin use as monotherapy is associated with the β-amyloid formation in elderly diabetic patients. In contrast to insulin, metformin had no role in degrading these harmful proteins. The researchers also found that metformin enhances the desirable effects of insulin when combined (63).

Vitamin B12 is known to be associated with dementia, but the association of metformin-induced B12 deficiency on cognitive impairment remain to be elucidated. A case-control study conducted in Australia (64) observed the negative effect of metformin on cognitive abilities. Furthermore, the investigators showed that these effects were B12 and calcium responsive. Although it was a case-control study with the relatively small size of the study sample, these results cannot be ignored. Another larger (more than fourteen thousand) population-based case-control study (65) stated that in contrast to sulfonylureas, thiazolidinediones, and insulin, metformin use in the long term is suggested to increase the risk of developing AD. A large cohort (66) (Participants=800,000) with long duration of follow-up conducted in Taiwan showed that both metformin and sulfonylureas reduced the risk of dementia, furthermore the combination of these drugs reduced the incidence by 35% over eight years.

A recent randomized controlled trial with a large sample and extended period of follow-up concluded that the term use of metformin in diabetes prevention program is not associated with cognitive impairment (67). Orkaby et al. (68) conducted a recent research among veterans ≥65 years, the study recruited more than 28,000 participants and controlled for various confounders, the researchers found that metformin was associated with lower rates of dementia than sulfonylureas.

Metformin, B12 deficiency, and cognitive impairment:

B12 deficiency can cause cognitive impairment; there is a small subset of neurodegenerative dementia that is reversible with B12 supplementation (69). The high dose of metformin but not the duration it has been shown to cause B12 deficiency (70), and the American Diabetes Association (6) recommended B12 estimation and correction when appropriate. Recent observational studies showed contradicting conclusions, while some (71) reported no association of metformin use with B12 deficiency, others (72) indicates a low level of metformin use. However, the relationship of metformin-induced B12 deficiency with cognitive impairment is uncertain. A case-control study (73) with small study sample showed no link between metformin-induced B12 deficiency and dementia. On the other hand, observational reviews (74) showed that B12 deficiency in patients with type 2 using metformin is associated with cognitive impairment and depression.

The following are proposed mechanisms for B12 deficiency due to metformin:

- Competitive inhibition or inactivation of Vitamin B12 absorption
- Interaction with the cubilinendocytic receptor
- Alterations in small bowel motility which stimulates bacterial overgrowth and subsequent Vitamin B12 deficiency
- Alterations in intrinsic factor (IF) levels
- Inhibition of the calcium-dependent absorption of Vitamin B12-IF complex at the terminal ileum. This inhibitory effect can be reversed with calcium supplementation.

Prospective analysis to study the association metformin-induced B12 deficiency and cognitive impairment are needed. Due to the current lack of a strong evidence linking metformin-induced B12 deficiency with cognitive impairment, and the fact that B12 deficiency can correct by simple routes (sublingually (75) or orally), state of the art is to check for B12 deficiency and correct as needed. The variation in the prevalence of metformin associated B12 deficiency is probably due to the different assay used and the variation in the cut-off values. The topic is further complicated by the yet undefined effects of the functional and marginal B12 deficiency (76).

Chapter 5. The intestinal microbiota and type 3 diabetes mellitus

The human intestine contains more than 100000 billion bacteria; various factors affect the composition of bacteria including age, geographical location, diet, exercise, weight, metabolic (formerly bariatric) surgery, and metformin. The bacteria play a vital role in insulin sensitivity and gut integrity. Although in its infancy, the composition of microbiota and the specific role in the promotion or prevention of diseases is in progress (Clostridium ramosum and Enterococcus cloacae versus bifidobacteria and Akkermansiamuciniphila (77,78)). Microbiota affects various organs, it had been shown that a cross-talk is present in the brain and the microbiota. It is interesting to note that children born by cesarean section are at a higher risk of type 2 diabetes due to altered gut microbiota.

Diabetes mellitus type 2 and AD are highly prevalent disease and are causes of much health concern. The diseases historically share the same molecular pathology, but the exact mechanisms remain to be elucidated. The significant attention raised due to the alarming increase of both type 2 &3 diabetes mellitus, the great socioeconomic burden, and the lack of precise early diagnostic methods for an effective therapy and prevention are reasons for innovative curative approaches including the bacteriophage and nanotechnology. The available drugs for the treatment of both type 2&3 diabetes mellitus have several limitations:

- They also give symptomatic relief from the basic pathophysiology and not curative or preventive, although type 2 diabetes complication can be delayed or prevented.
- The limited efficacy due failure of delivery including crossing of the blood-brain barrier

- Lack of target specificity. A good example is the action of insulin on both the metabolic and mitogenic pathways leading to glycemic control at the expense of possible increasing malignancy
- Diminished potency of some drugs (79)

Bacteriophage:

The fact that wound infection by resistant bacteria among patients with diabetes is the most frequent cause of non-traumatic amputation, the lack of efficacy of antibiotic alone to heal the infected wound, and the need to the immunomodulation of anti-amyloid beta peptide response in AD, have led to the introduction of bacteriophage as a novel approach in the management of diabetes wound infection and Alzheimer's disease. Phages are viruses infecting bacteria without the ability to infect mammalian cell, so limited side effects. With improving the delivery system, bacteriophage can be used in the treatment of AD and prevention diabetes wound infection in combination with an antibiotic (80).

Microbiota, immune system, and neuroendocrine:

Recent animal studies (81) showed that mtDNA mutations lead to substantial differences in the composition of gut microbial communities. Such a differences could be the base of metabolic diseases and if targeted could be a potential therapeutic approach. Human evolution within a microbial ecology leads to physiological interlinking; a good example is the brain cross-talk with gut microbiota through the immune system. The gut hormone through the vagus nerve, tryptophan metabolism, and the products of microbiota could influence brain development, behavior, and functions. Furthermore, gut microbiota is suggested to have a role in shaping cognitive networks encompassing emotional and social domains in neurodevelopmental disorders (82). A recent study published in Nature (83) conducted in mice to induce colitis by intrarectal injection of 2,4,6-trinitrobenzenesulfonic acid (TNBS) observed following were in mice:

- ✓ Increased gut permeability

- ✓ Increased fecal and blood levels of lipopolysaccharide (LPS)

- ✓ Increased number of Enterobacteriaceae, particularly Escherichia coli (EC)

- ✓ Decreased level of Lactobacillus johnsonii (LJ)

- ✓ Cognitive impairment. Furthermore, treatment of mice with E coli isolated from mice with colitis leads to the above-unwanted effects which were reversed by Lactobacillus johnsonii (LJ) treatment.

Previous studies pointed that, the interaction between the fetus and the vaginal microbes is essential for the development of gut microbiota which in turn mediates the cross-talk between the immune system and neuroendocrine system to maintain homeostasis. The exact mechanism remains elusive. The main challenge is to fully decipher the molecular mechanisms that link these systems in a network of communication to eventually translate these findings to the human situation, both in health and disease (84,85). Furthermore, microbiota was suggested to play an important role in the development of postnatal gastrointestinal functions during the early colonization of the host. Although a big gap remained to be filled, the interaction between stress, gut microbiota, activation of pre-sensitized T lymphocytes in a genetically predisposed individual is crucial for tissue damage and neurodegeneration (86). Gaining knowledge of the cross talk between components of the gut microbiota - an immune system in particular T -lymphocytes and the brain could be beneficial in the design of future therapeutic approaches. There is an accumulative evidence that a feedback exists between the hypothalamus-pituitary-adrenal axis and the gut. Through the gut microbiota and other intestinal substances such as catecholamines and γ-aminobutyric acid. The microbiota can affect the development of this endocrine axis and a positive feedback through which the hypothalamic-pituitary axis increase the bacterial proliferative capacity and pathogenicity (87,88). The metabolite signals of the gut microbiota to distant organs in a mammal is essential to maintain the vital functions. However, the gut microbiota has been associated with some diseases including Alzheimer,s disease (type 3 diabetes mellitus) (89).

Gut microbiota and Alzheimer's disease:

Gut microbiota imbalance is associated with obesity and low-grade inflammation that increase the risk of developing type 2&3 diabetes mellitus. The cause of AD is a matter of debate, but there is a growing body of evidence suggesting that obesity is associated with:

- Alteration of gut microbiota
- An altered representation of microbiota genes
- Reduced bacterial diversity, and metabolic pathways
- Change within the diversity of microbiota that also predisposes to diabetes mellitus which has a direct relation to AD pathogenesis (90).

It has been suggested that certain diets in a genetically predisposed individual and alteration of gut microbiota lead to low-grade inflammation and disruption of the intestinal barrier. The ultimate result is obesity and insulin resistance. Thus it is proposed that gut microbiota alteration contributes to the development of type 2,3 &1 diabetes mellitus (91).

Metformin (*Galegaofficinalis, French lilac, goat's rue*) **effects on microbiota:**

Metformin plays an important role in energy balance through the activation of AMP-activated protein kinase (AMPK) and down-regulation of several pathways. By decreasing the ATP production and increasing consumption, the balance of AMP/ATP is maintained. Previous literature showed that metformin regulation of gluconeogenesis and hyperglycemia independent of AMPK, suggesting that metformin-induced improvement of metabolic disorders is associated with the energy state of the body (92-96). The observation that intravenous metformin does not improve glucose metabolism suggests that other organs like gastrointestinal tract plays a crucial role in metformin action. Glucagon-like peptide-1 (GLP-1), peptide tyrosine-tyrosine (PYY), secreted by the enteroendocrine cells in the gut, and changes in the gut microbial community were all suggested (96). Metformin enters the hepatocytes by organic cation transporter-1 (OCT-1) transporter, and there it is thought to alter mitochondrial function and AMP kinase. The following section will discuss the role of metformin in the regulation of microbiota, energy balance, obesity, and type 2 &3 diabetes mellitus.

Animal studies showed that metformin similar to berberine shifted the overall structure of intestinal microbiota. Furthermore the drugs showed reverting effects on high fat diet-induced structural changes on microbiome and reduced the diversity of this abundant gut bacteria. Berberine and metformin to a lesser extent have increased the organisms related to the putative short-chain fatty acids including: Allobaculum, Bacteroides, Blautia, Butyricoccus, and Phascolarctobacterium. By contrast the drugs reduced other operational taxonomic units (OTUs) related to obesity phenotypes changes (endotoxin-producing bacteria and sulfate-reducing bacteria including Escherichia coli and Desulfovibrio sp). Up to 30% of the orally administered metformin is not absorbed and exerts its effects on the gut microbiota and the rest is absorbed to take its actions. Metformin is effective in a wide range of diseases including aging, cardiovascular disease Non-Alcoholic Fatty Liver Disease, Polycystic ovary syndrome, and even cancer, a reasonable explanation for metformin to be effective in such a wide disorders is through its effects on microbiota. Indeed microbiota has been shown to play a role in all of the aforementioned disorders. It is interesting to note that transfer of microbiota from toll-like receptor 5 (a innate immune component that is abundant in the gut and help to fight against infection) deficient mice, with hyperphagia and metabolic syndrome, into a wild-type germfree mice conferred most of the metabolic phenotypes to the recipients, including hyperphagia(97,98) suggesting a role of microbiota in food intake regulation. The previous study also expressed the importance of the immune system in microbiota balance and the development of metabolic features including obesity, diabetes, and dyslipidemia. The interaction between the gut microbiota and the host and the different species is complex. The host provide a shelter with nutrients for the gut flora, on the other hands the microbiota facilitates host adaptation by enabling e.g., immunomodulation, vitamin synthesis, gastrointestinal maturation, detoxification, and xenobiotic. Thus the relation is holoboint, but sometimes the microbiome acts as pathogenic or commensal (99). The nematode Caenorhabditiselegans is unique in that only one species is present as a food source under certain culture conditions.Escherichia coli is suggested to play a major role in C. elegans metabolism and nutrition than merely being a source of food, and sometimes it acts as microbiota (100). Cabreiro et al. (99) in their experimental study on C. elegans showed that, metformin effects in increasing the lifespan of this nematode by inhibiting E. coli folate and methionine metabolism and regulation of eating. Metformin has direct toxic effects on metformin sensitive organisms (shorten lifespan) and indirect effects (increase lifespan). Furthermore the effects are species dependent (in the absence of E. coli or the drug-resistant organism there was no effects). The presence of a huge number of gut microbiota, the variation between the same species, the interaction with other gastrointestinal commensals, the section of the proper metabolic pathway in the causation of a specific disease to be targeted by the right interventions are major challenges along the world of microbiota. The possible interaction between the skin (the larger organ in humans), and the respiratory systems complicate the matter further. A study (101) using multi-country T2D metagenomic dataset and controlled for disease and other drugs supported the microbiota mediated therapeutic effects of metformin by short chain fatty acid and butyrate producing taxa. Furthermore, the researchers showed that the unwanted side effects of metformin could be mediated by E. coli relative abundance. Alteration in the enterohepatic circulation of bile acids, changes in gut hormones especially GLP-1, and the modulation of microbiota after oral administration of metformin pointed to the importance of the gastrointestinal tract including neuroendocrine cells and hormones, and the abundant world of microbiome with its interactions and diversity in the action of metformin and pathophysiology of various metabolic and neurodegenerative disorders (102).

Metformin has been found to inhibit dehydrogenase, resulting in the reduced conversion of lactate and glycerol to glucose. The inhibition of this enzyme in microbiota and accumulation of lactic acid in the gut together with methane with the end product of branched-chain amino acid, and bile acids leads to nausea, diarrhea, and heartburn in (47.4%),(62.1%), and (52.1%) respectively. Five percents of patients on metformin discontinue metformin due to these events. The inhibition of dehydrogenase could also lead to the rare serious lactic acidosis. A study used Inulin

(3.79 g) from agave, beta-glucan (2.03 g) from oats and polyphenols from blueberry pomace collectively known as GIMM (NM504) and regarded as safe by Federal Drug Administration (FDA) showed that this product when combined with metformin in patients with diabetes, the gastrointestinal side effects were well-tolerated. Furthermore, the fasting plasma glucose improved substantially in patients taking the combination therapy than those taking metformin alone. The GIMM (NM504) diet acts by:

- ✓ Retard absorption of small molecules by increasing the viscosity of luminal contents
- ✓ Fortify the mucosal barrier, sequester bile acids and salts, and deliver a potent antioxidant to combat the increased demand for oxidative stress.
- ✓ Stimulate blooms of competing for commensal microbiota that generate short-chain fatty acids (SCFA) instead of lactic acid (103).

Metformin Metabolism:

- ❖ Immediate release is absorbed mainly in small intestine (negligible in stomach and large intestine)
- ❖ Intravenous administration of metformin results in rapid renal elimination, with little or no metformin detectable in the feces.
- ❖ Metformin MR (modified-release) uses a dual polymer matrix to delay the transit and slow the release of metformin in the gut to increase tolerability.
- ❖ Metformin DR (delayed-release) had lower bioavailability but retaining its glucose-lowering effects compared to extended release and immediate release.
- ❖ Metformin uptake is saturable and dose-dependent, many receptors including cation transporters, serotonin, and MATE transporters.

❖ Metformin increases GLP-1 secretion, decrease histamine and serotonin metabolism with minimal effects on DPP4.

❖ Metformin increase glucose transport and metabolism in the gut increasing lactate

❖ It affects bile acid absorption and increase butyrate producing bacteria

❖ Metformin acts through the vagus nerve and nucleus of the solitary tract to increase intestinal gluconeogenesis and decrease the same process in the liver reducing glucose in the blood (104-107).

The combination of metformin and H. cordata enriched with flavonoid and phenolic ingredients have been shown to improve hyperlipidemia, insulin sensitivity, and reduce inflammation and endotoxinemia possibly through microbiota regulation in particular Gram-negative bacteria, *Roseburia*, and *Akkermansia*.. so this combination could be an efficient approach in the treatment of patients with the metabolic syndrome (108).

Chapter 6. Probiotics, gut microbiota, and Alzheimer's disease

Plenty of evidence exists about the role of probiotics in improving the nervous system function. A controlled trial conducted in diabetic and healthy rats fed either normal diet or diet plus probiotics showed that probiotics efficiently reverse diabetes-related cognitive disturbances and their proposed synaptic mechanisms and restoring deteriorated brain functions (109).

amyloid-β and tau pathology (the bases of extracellular neurofibrillary tangles) begin around the age of 40 but need more 20years to translate into cognitive impairment. Once the AD is clinically manifested, it is far more late for treatment to be efficient high lightening the importance of the earlier introduction of lifestyle and dietary changes (110,111).

Probiotics (living microorganisms) confer the following benefits when introduced optimally in the host (112):

- ✓ immunomodulatory functions (113)
- ✓ prevention of infections (114)
- ✓ improvement of the intestinal environment
- ✓ Anti-obesity effects (115)
- ✓ Cancer prevention, and lifespan extension (116,117)

Interestingly, some probiotics can influence the microbiota brain axis with indirect effects on the central nervous system and behavior (118). Previous literature (119) reported the positive effects of probiotics on anxiety provoked by early life stress and reduced inflammation, also a mixture of probiotic-containing seven gram-positive bacteria was found to modulate neuronal functions and long-term potentiation in young and aged rats and could alter inflammation and neural plasticity in the brain through gene expression (120). Moreover probiotics mixture were found to affect the metabolic status and cognitive function in Alzheimer's disease (121).

There is increasing evidence that probiotics not only modulating the immunological and physiological function but may also alter brain function opening the road for effective interventions to a wider range of psychiatric and neurological diseases including the AD. It is observed that ICV infusion of Aβ in the rodent brain can mimic aspects of Alzheimer's disease and can be useful for developing and evaluating potential new therapies for this prevalent morbid disease (122, 123).

A recent animal study (118), showed the ICV injection of Aβ unregulated the genes involved in immune response and response to external stimuli in the hippocampus, thus reshaping gene expression. The researchers found that the above genes are normally expressed in the hippocampus of *B. breve* A1-administered mice indicating that this probiotic normalized the gene expression profile and suppressed the toxicity induced by Aβ. The study hypothesize that administration of *B. breve* A1 prevented cognitive decline in AD model mice through its modulating effect on the immune response and neuronal inflammation. It has been suggested that the gut microbiota composition is altered by probiotics which could affect module gene expression in the brain (120).Kobayashi et al. (118) in his animal study did not observe any marked short effect of *B. breve* A1 administration on the gut microbiota population and suggested that other mechanisms including the vagus nerve feedback on the brain could mediate probiotics effects on the brain gene expression. The vagus nerve has been shown to convey information from peripheral organs to the brain through acetylcholine. Probiotics have been shown to modulate anxiety-like behavior through the vagus nerve integrity. Furthermore, the vagus nerve stimulation has been suggested to exerts anti-inflammatory effects via the neurotransmitter acetylcholine (124-126).

Other than acetylcholine, metabolites generated by probiotics effects on the gut microbiota populations can cross the blood-brain barrier and affect neurocognitive functions, it is stated that (118) the administration of *B. breve* A1 A1 increased plasma acetate levels. Furthermore, the addition of acetate to drinking water resulted in partial cognitive improvement in Alzheimer's disease in mice. The mechanism of how acetate ameliorates memory dysfunction in AD mice is a place for future studies. Alzheimer's disease is classified in preclinical and clinical disease, the progression of Aβ induced inflammation, immunomodulation, and expression of genes in the hippocampus needs to be targeted in its early phase or before development in at-risk patients. The recognition of the specific pathways for AD development and the selection of safe effective interventions are priorities to fight this costly spreading disease. The phosphorylated tau protein pathway and the extracellular deposition of neurofibrillary tangles in another attractive field for research in the field of the AD, selection of animals reflecting the biological processes of the AD as traditional APP-overexpression mouse or APP knock-in mouse are important in the future research. Probiotic treatment could also improve the negative effects of diets on the gut bacterial composition and hence the prevention of endotoxinemia and low-grade inflammation that lead to insulin resistance, gene expression alteration, amyloid deposition, and neurocognitive dysfunction (127-129).

The Western diet, Alzheimer's disease, and probiotics:

Western diet has been linked to gut microbiome alteration and cognitive impairment including:

- ☒ Reduced short-chain fatty acids production, compromised barrier integrity
- ☒ Peripheral and central insulin receptor resistance
- ☒ Neuroinflammation

Endotoxemia promoted by WD, which is linked to cognitive impairment via translocation of gram-negative bacteria translocation into circulation, or the impairment permeability of the gut barrier. Both the Western Diet and gut microbiota intake have been shown to impair the permeability of the BBB. However, the mechanisms remain to be elucidated. Microbiota alterations by probiotics impair peripheral insulin sensitivity, which is strongly linked with central insulin resistance and hippocampal dysfunction. Furthermore, insulin protects against peripheral inflammatory responses to endotoxin and could prevent the deleterious effects imparted by Western diet (129).

Periodontitis, and type 2 &3 diabetes mellitus:

Periodontitis is a common and treatable disease that has been linked to both type 2 diabetes and AD. The endotoxinemia, peripheral insulin resistance, and neuroinflammation seem to be involved. Furthermore, anaerobes that cause periodontitis and Spirochetes were also associated with neurocognitive alterations.

The early detection and introduction of management are vital to prevent systemic infection and cognitive dysfunction (130).

Fecal transplantation (Bacteriotherapy, microbiota transplantation):

Is the administration of a fecal solution from a donor into the intestinal tract of a recipient. Microbiota is located in the skin, nose, mouth, guts, and genitals. In the beginning, it was restricted to patients with recurrent Clostridium difficile resistant to standard therapy. Recently the treatment extended to include many diseases including obesity and the metabolic syndrome. The transplantation is usually performed by colonoscopy, nasogastric tube, or retention enema. An oral capsule is introduced recently. Consent is vital; counseling should be offered to the recipient. The donor must be known to the patient and should be investigated carefully for stool and blood infection transmission (131-132).

Conclusions:

Lactate a metabolite of glucose is essential for neuronal metabolism, the expression of genes involved in memory, and the formation of dendrites and synapses.The disruption of the physiological balance could result in metabolic compromise leading to diabetes including type-3 diabetes. Insulin resistance plays a crucial role in the development of amyloid β and neurofibrillary tangles (the bases of the AD). Many antihyperglycemic drugs including metformin, intranasal insulin, pioglitazone, GLP-1 agonists, DPP-4 inhibitors, Glimepiride, and glipizide are promising approaches for type 3 diabetes management. GLP-1 agonists are very promising due to efficacy, no problem with dosing, and they readily cross the blood-brain barrier. Both animal and human studies conducted on metformin and AD are contradicting with some showed the association of metformin with the AD, and others showed that metformin improved improve cognition, while others were neutral. In the face of contradicting observation regarding the role of metformin-induced B12 deficiency and cognitive impairment, the recommendation is to check for B12 deficiency and replace orally or sublingually. Although the combination of drugs is more efficacious, the current medications used in the treatment of type 3 diabetes mellitus have many limitations including that they are symptomatic treatment, lack of efficacy due to delivery failure including the crossing of the blood-brain barrier, diminished potency of some, and most importantly Lack of target specificity. A cross-talk exists between the gut and microbiota, brain, liver, and hypothalomopituitary axis. Metformin exerts its action in part through the production of lactate in the gut, increasing the butyrate producing microbiota, and reduction of E. coli. The lactate produced by microbiota and metformin could be involved in the gastrointestinal side effects in spite of the beneficial effects on the brain. Combination of therapies with different modalities of action could be more efficacious in the treatment of AD, and the enhancing the side effects of metformin. Probiotics are emerging as an important therapy in Alzheimers disease, and the fecal transplantation could be far in the horizon in its management.

Recommendations:

- More research is needed to address the specific pathophysiology of type 3 diabetes to implement specific intervention in both type 2 &3 diabetes mellitus

- A great effort is needed to fully decipher the crosstalk between the gut microbiota as a novel therapy for metabolic diseases and various organs including the brain

- The gut barrier, and the blood-brain barrier and the role of the vagus nerve as stimulator effecter between the gut, liver, and brain are attractive for future research.

- Longitudinal studies on humans are needed to assess newer combination therapy for the treatment of AD

- The early detection of periodontitis to prevent systemic inflammation and endotoxinemia and hence AD

Abbreviations:

AD: Alzheimer's disease

Aβ: Amyloid beta

NFTs: Neurofibrillary tangles

LXRs: liver X receptors

PPARγ: Peroxisome-proliferator receptor γ

TOMM40 gene: Translocase of outer mitochondrial membrane 40 homolog gene

GLP-1: Glucagon like peptide

PI 3-K: Phosphoinositide 3-kinase

Akt: Protein kinase B

AMPK: AMP-activated protein kinase

ACE-Is: Angiotensin-converting enzyme inhibitors

LPS: lipopolysaccharide

LJ: Lactobacillus johnsonii

EC: Escherichia coli

PYY: Peptide tyrosine-tyrosine

OCT-1: Organic cation transporter-1

OTUs: Operational taxonomic units

SCFA: Short-chain fatty acids

WD: Western Diet

References:

1. World Health Organization. Dementia [article online] 2012. Available from HTTP://www.who.int/mediacentre/factsheets/fs362/en/. Accessed 13 February 2015

2. Prince M, Bryce R, Albanese E, Wimo A, Ribeiro W, Ferri CP. The global prevalence of dementia: a systematic review and metaanalysis. Alzheimers Dement. 2013 Jan;9(1):63-75.e2. doi: 10.1016/j.jalz.2012.11.007

3. Chatterjee S, Peters SA, Woodward M, Mejia Arango S, Batty GD, Beckett N et al. Type 2 Diabetes as
a Risk Factor for Dementia in Women Compared With Men:
A Pooled Analysis of 2.3 Million People Comprising More Than 100,000 Cas
es of Dementia. Diabetes Care. 2016 Feb;39(2):300-7. doi: 10.2337/dc15-1588. Epub 2015 Dec 17.

4. Rizvi SM, Shaikh S, Waseem SM, Shakil S, Abuzenadah AM, Biswas D, Tabrez S, Ashraf GM, Kamal MA. Role of anti-diabetic drugs as therapeutic agents in Alzheimer's disease.EXCLI J. 2015 May 19;14:684-96. doi: 10.17179/excli2015-252. eCollection 2015

5. Fradkin JE, Rodgers GP. Glycemic therapy for type 2 diabetes: Choices Expand, Data Lag Behind. Ann Intern Med. 2017 Feb 21;166(4):309-310. doi: 10.7326/M16-2883. Epub 2017 Jan 3.

6. American Diabetes Association Standards of Medical Care in Diabetes. Lifestyle Management Diabetes Care 2017;40(Suppl. 1):S33–S43 | DOI: 10.2337/dc17-S007

7. Khattar D, Khaliq F, Vaney N[1], Madhu SV. Is Metformin-Induced Vitamin B12 Deficiency Responsible for Cognitive Decline in Type 2 Diabetes?.

Indian J Psychol Med. 2016 Jul-Aug;38(4):285-90. doi: 10.4103/0253-7176.185952.

8. Biemans E, Hart HE, Rutten GE, Cuellar Renteria VG, Kooijman-Buiting AM, Beulens JW. Cobalamin status and its relation with depression, cognition and neuropathy in patients with type 2 diabetes mellitus using metformin. ActaDiabetol. 2015 Apr;52(2):383-93. doi: 10.1007/s00592-014-0661-4. Epub 2014 Oct 15.

9. Ye F, Luo YJ, Xiao J, Yu NW, Yi G. Impact of Insulin Sensitizers on the Incidence of Dementia: A Meta-Analysis.Dement GeriatrCognDisord. 2016;41(5-6):251-60. doi: 10.1159/000445941. Epub 2016 Jun 2.

10. Allard JS, Perez EJ, Fukui K, Carpenter P, Ingram DK, de Cabo R. Prolonged metformin treatment leads to reduced transcription of Nrf2 and neurotrophic factors without cognitive impairment in older C57BL/6J mice. Behav Brain Res. 2016 Mar 15;301:1-9. doi: 10.1016/j.bbr.2015.12.012. Epub 2015 Dec 14.

11. Daviglus ML, Bell CC, Berrettini W, Bowen PE, Connolly ES, Cox NJ, Dunbar-Jacob JM, Granieri EC, Hunt G, McGarry K, et al. National Institutes of Health state-of-the-science conference statement: preventing Alzheimer disease and cognitive decline. Ann Intern Med 2010;153:176–81.

12. Alzheimer's SocietyAlzheimer's Society online information—About dementia—What is dementia? Leading the fight against Dementia [Internet]. 2014 [cited 2016 Mar 30]. Available from: http://www.alzheimers.org.uk/site/scripts/documents.php?categoryID=200360.

13. Tricco AC, Soobiah C, Berliner S, Ho JM, Ng CH, Ashoor HM, Chen MH, Hemmelgarn BSS. Efficacy and safety of cognitive enhancers for patients with mild cognitive impairment: a systematic review and meta-analysis. CMAJ 2013;185:1393–401.

14. González-Reyes RE[1], Aliev G, Ávila-Rodrigues M, Barreto GE. Alterations in Glucose Metabolism on Cognition: A Possible Link Between Diabetes and Dementia. Curr Pharm Des. 2016;22(7):812-8.

15. Kang S, Lee YH, Lee JE. Metabolism-Centric Overview of the Pathogenesis of Alzheimer's Disease.Yonsei Med J. 2017 May;58(3):479-488. doi: 10.3349/ymj.2017.58.3.479.

16. Leszek J, Trypka E, Tarasov VV, Ashraf GM, AlievG.Type 3 Diabetes Mellitus: A Novel Implication of Alzheimers Disease.Curr Top Med Chem. 2017;17(12):1331-1335. doi: 10.2174/1568026617666170103163403.

17. Kandimalla R, Thirumala V, Reddy PH.
Is Alzheimer's disease a Type 3 Diabetes? A critical appraisal.
BiochimBiophysActa. 2017 May;1863(5):1078-1089. doi: 10.1016/j.bbadis.2016.08.018. Epub 2016 Aug 25.

18. Hazar N, Seddigh L, Rampisheh Z, Nojomi M. Population attributable fraction of modifiable risk factors for Alzheimer disease: A systematic review of systematic reviews. Iran J Neurol. 2016 Jul 6;15(3):164-72.

19. Petersson SD[1], Philippou E. Mediterranean Diet, Cognitive Function, and Dementia: A Systematic Review of the Evidence. AdvNutr. 2016 Sep 15;7(5):889-904. doi: 10.3945/an.116.012138. Print 2016 Sep.

20. Walker JM, Harrison FE. Shared Neuropathological Characteristics of Obesity, Type 2 Diabetes and Alzheimer's Disease: Impacts on Cognitive Decline.Nutrients. 2015 Sep 1;7(9):7332-57. doi: 10.3390/nu7095341

21. Li X, Song D, Leng SX. Link between type 2 diabetes and Alzheimer's disease: from epidemiology to mechanism and treatment.ClinInterv Aging. 2015 Mar 10;10:549-60. doi: 10.2147/CIA.S74042. eCollection 2015.

22. Risner M, Saunders A, Altman J, et al. Efficacy of rosiglitazone in a genetically defined population with mild-to-moderate Alzheimer's disease. Pharmacogenomics J. 2006;6(4):246–254.

23. . Bomfim TR, Forny-Germano L, Sathler LB, et al. An anti-diabetes agent protects the mouse brain from defective insulin signaling caused by Alzheimer's disease–associated Aβ oligomers. J Clin Invest. 2012;122(4):1339–1353.

24. Skerrett R, Pellegrino MP, Casali BT, Taraboanta L, Landreth GE. Combined Liver X Receptor/Peroxisome Proliferator-activated Receptor γ Agonist Treatment Reduces Amyloid β Levels and Improves Behavior in Amyloid Precursor Protein/Presenilin 1 Mice.J Biol Chem. 2015 Aug 28;290(35):21591-602. doi: 10.1074/jbc.M115.652008. Epub 2015 Jul 10.

25. Miller BW, Willett KC, Desilets AR. Rosiglitazone and pioglitazone for the treatment of Alzheimer's disease. Ann Pharmacother. 2011 Nov;45(11):1416-24. doi: 10.1345/aph.1Q238. Epub 2011 Oct 25.

26. Sato T, Hanyu H, Hirao K, Kanetaka H, Sakurai H, Iwamoto T. Efficacy of PPAR-γ agonist pioglitazone in mild Alzheimer disease.

NeurobiolAging. 2011 Sep;32(9):1626-33. doi: 10.1016/j.neurobiolaging.2009.10.009. Epub 2009 Nov 17.

27. Cheng H, Shang Y, Jiang L, Shi TL, Wang L. The peroxisome proliferators activated receptor-gamma agonists as therapeutics for the treatment of Alzheimer's disease and mild-to-moderate Alzheimer's disease: a meta-analysis.Int J Neurosci. 2016;126(4):299-307. doi: 10.3109/00207454.2015.1015722. Epub 2015 May 22.

28. Liu J, Wang LN, Jia JP. Peroxisome proliferator-activated receptor-gamma agonists for Alzheimer's disease and amnestic mild cognitive impairment: a systematic review and meta-analysis. Drugs Aging. 2015 Jan;32(1):57-65. doi: 10.1007/s40266-014-0228-7.

29. Galea E, Feinstein DL, Lacombe P. Pioglitazone does not increase cerebral glucose utilisation in a murine model of Alzheimer's disease and decreases it in wild-type mice. Diabetologia. 2006 Sep;49(9):2153-61. Epub 2006 Jul 8.

30. Nicolakakis N, Aboulkassim T, Ongali B, Lecrux C, Fernandes P, Rosa-Neto P, Tong XK, Hamel E. Complete rescue of cerebrovascular function in aged Alzheimer's disease transgenic mice by antioxidants and pioglitazone, a peroxisome proliferator-activated receptor gamma agonist. J Neurosci. 2008 Sep 10;28(37):9287-96. doi: 10.1523/JNEUROSCI.3348-08.2008.

31. Fessel WJ. Concordance of Several Subcellular Interactions Initiates Alzheimer's Dementia: Their Reversal Requires Combination Treatment. Am J Alzheimers Dis Other Demen. 2017 May;32(3):166-181. doi: 10.1177/1533317517698790. Epub 2017 Mar 17.

32. Geldmacher DS, Fritsch T, McClendon MJ, Landreth G. A randomized pilot clinical trial of the safety of pioglitazone in treatment of patients with Alzheimer disease. Archives of neurology. 2011;68(1):45–50.

33. Sato T, Hanyu H, Hirao K, Kanetaka H, Sakurai H, Iwamoto T. Efficacy of PPAR-gamma agonist pioglitazone in mild Alzheimer disease. Neurobiology of aging. 2011;32(9):1626–33.

34. Health USNIo. Biomarker Qualification for Risk of Mild Cognitive Impairment (MCI) Due to Alzheimer's Disease (AD) and Safety and Efficacy of Pioglitazone in Delaying Its Onset. 2014 Jul 24; Available from: http://clinicaltrials.gov/show/NCT01931566.

35. Hsu D[1], Marshall GA. Primary and Secondary Prevention Trials in Alzheimer Disease: Looking Back, Moving Forward. Curr Alzheimer Res. 2017;14(4):426-440. doi: 10.2174/1567205013666160930112125.

36. McClean PL, Parthsarathy V, Faivre E, Hölscher C. The diabetes drug liraglutide prevents degenerative processes in a mouse model of Alzheimer's disease. J Neurosci. 2011;31(17):6587–6594.

37. Adler BL, Yarchoan M, Hwang HM, Louneva N, Blair JA, Palm R, et al. Casadesus G Neuroprotective effects of the amylin analogue pramlintide on Alzheimer's disease pathogenesis and cognition. Neurobiol Aging. 2014;35:793–801

38. Potes CS, Boyle CN, Wookey PJ, Riediger T, Lutz TA. Involvement of the extracellular signal-regulated kinase 1/2 signaling pathway in amylin's eating inhibitory effect. Am J PhysiolRegulIntegr Comp Physiol. 2012;302:340–351.

39. Farret A, Lugo-Garcia L, Galtier F, Gross R, Petit P. Pharmacological interventions that directly stimulate or modulate insulin secretion from pancreatic
beta-cell: implications for the treatment of type 2
diabetes. FundamClinPharmacol. 2005;19:647–656.

40. Isik AT, Soysal P, Yay A, UsarelC.The effects of sitagliptin, a DPP-4
inhibitor, on cognitive functions in elderly diabetic patients with or without
Alzheimer's disease.Diabetes Res ClinPract. 2017 Jan;123:192-198. doi:
10.1016/j.diabres.2016.12.010. Epub 2016 Dec 21.

41. Matsushita T, Yajima K, Sumitomo H, Shigeta M, Nishimura K, Shirabe
S, Sakai M, Katayama T, Kanno K, Sakurai H, Nakano T, Kitaoka M, Ueki A.
[A questionnaire survey on current status of anti-diabetic therapy for diabetic
patients with dementia].Nihon Ronen IgakkaiZasshi. 2013;50(2):219-26.
Article in Japanese]

42. Fukuen S, Iwaki M, Yasui A, Makishima M, Matsuda M, Shimomura I.
Sulfonylurea agents exhibit peroxisome proliferator-activated receptor gamma
agonistic activity. J Biol Chem. 2005;280:23653–23659.

43. Scarsi M, Podvinec M, Roth A, Hug H, Kersten S, Albrecht H, et al.
Sulfonylureas and glinides exhibit peroxisome proliferator-activated receptor
gamma activity: a combined virtual screening and biological assay
approach. MolPharmacol. 2007;71:398–406.

44. Mahboobi H, Golmirzaei J, Gan SH, Jalalian M, Kamal MA. Humanin: a
possible linkage between Alzheimer's disease and type 2 diabetes.CNS
NeurolDisord Drug Targets. 2014 Apr;13(3):543-52.

45. Jha NK, Jha SK, Kumar D, Kejriwal N, Sharma R, Ambasta RK, Kumar P.
Impact of Insulin Degrading Enzyme and

Neprilysinin Alzheimer's Disease Biology: Characterization of Putative

Cognates for Therapeutic Applications.J Alzheimers Dis. 2015;48(4):891-917.

doi: 10.3233/JAD-150379.

46. Maiese K. Novel nervous and multi-system regenerative therapeutic strategies

for diabetes mellitus with mTOR.Neural Regen Res. 2016 Mar;11(3):372-85.

doi: 10.4103/1673-5374.179032.

47. Rygiel K. Can angiotensin-converting enzyme inhibitors impact cognitive

decline in early stages of Alzheimer's disease? An overview of research

evidence in the elderly patient population.J Postgrad Med. 2016 Oct-

Dec;62(4):242-248. doi: 10.4103/0022-3859.188553.

48. Talbot K, Wang HY, Kazi H, Han LY, Bakshi KP, Stucky A, et al.

Demonstrated brain insulin resistance in Alzheimer's disease patients is

associated with IGF-1 resistance, IRS-1 dysregulation, and cognitive decline. J

Clin Invest. 2012;122:1316–38. doi: 10.1172/JCI59903.

49. Barini E, Antico O, Zhao Y, Asta F, Tucci V, Catelani T, Marotta R, Xu

H, Gasparini L. Metformin promotes tau aggregation and exacerbates

abnormal behavior in a mouse model of tauopathy.MolNeurodegener. 2016

Feb 9;11:16. doi: 10.1186/s13024-016-0082-7.

50. Yarchoan M, Toledo JB, Lee EB, Arvanitakis Z, Kazi H, Han LY, et al.

Abnormal serine phosphorylation of insulin receptor substrate 1 is associated

with tau pathology in Alzheimer's disease and

tauopathies. ActaNeuropathol. 2014;128:679–89. doi: 10.1007/s00401-014-

1328-5.

51. Viollet B, Guigas B, Sanz Garcia N, Leclerc J, Foretz M, Andreelli F. Cellular and molecular mechanisms of metformin: an overview. Clin Sci. 2012;122:253–70. doi: 10.1042/CS20110386.

52. Hundal RS, Krssak M, Dufour S, Laurent D, Lebon V, Chandramouli V, et al. Mechanism by which metformin reduces glucose production in type 2 diabetes. Diabetes. 2000;49:2063–9. doi: 10.2337/diabetes.49.12.2063.

53. Picone P, Vilasi S, Librizzi F, Contardi M, Nuzzo D, Caruana L, Baldassano S, Amato A[4], Mulè F, San Biagio PL, Giacomazza D, Di Carlo M. Biological and biophysics aspects of metformin-induced effects: cortex mitochondrial dysfunction and promotion of toxic amyloid pre-fibrillar aggregates.Aging (Albany NY). 2016 Aug;8(8):1718-34. doi: 10.18632/aging.101004.

54. Son SM, Shin HJ, Byun J, Kook SY, Moon M, Chang YJ, Mook-Jung I. Metformin Facilitates Amyloid-β Generation by β- and γ-Secretases via Autophagy Activation.J Alzheimers Dis. 2016;51(4):1197-208. doi: 10.3233/JAD-151200.

55. Picone P, Nuzzo D[1], Caruana L, Messina E, Barera A, Vasto S, Di Carlo M. Metformin increases APP expression and processing via oxidative stress, mitochondrial dysfunction and NF-κB activation: Use of insulin to attenuate metformin's effect.BiochimBiophysActa. 2015 May;1853(5):1046-59. doi: 10.1016/j.bbamcr.2015.01.017. Epub 2015 Feb 7.

56. McNeilly AD, Williamson R, Balfour DJ, Stewart CA, Sutherland C. A high-fat-diet-induced cognitive deficit in rats that is not prevented by improving insulin sensitivity with metformin. Diabetologia. 2012 Nov;55(11):3061-70. doi: 10.1007/s00125-012-2686-y. Epub 2012 Aug 18.

57. Chen B, Teng Y, Zhang X, Lv X, Yin Y. Metformin Alleviated Aβ-Induced Apoptosis via the Suppression of JNK MAPK Signaling Pathway in Cultured Hippocampal Neurons. Biomed Res Int. 2016;2016:1421430. doi: 10.1155/2016/1421430. Epub 2016 Jun 15.

58. Chiang MC, Cheng YC, Chen SJ, Yen CH, Huang RN. Metformin activation of AMPK-dependent pathways is neuroprotective in human neural stem cells against Amyloid-beta-induced mitochondrial dysfunction.Exp Cell Res. 2016 Oct 1;347(2):322-31. doi: 10.1016/j.yexcr.2016.08.013. Epub 2016 Aug 21.

59. Kickstein E, Krauss S, Thornhill P, Rutschow D, Zeller R, Sharkey J, Williamson R, Fuchs M, Köhler A, Glossmann H, Schneider R, Sutherland C, Schweiger S.Biguanide metformin acts on tau phosphorylation via mTOR/protein phosphatase 2A (PP2A) signaling. ProcNatlAcadSci U S A. 2010 Dec 14;107(50):21830-5. doi: 10.1073/pnas.0912793107. Epub 2010 Nov 22.

60. Asadbegi M, Yaghmaei P, Salehi I, Ebrahim-Habibi A, Komaki A. Neuroprotective effects of metformin against Aβ-mediated inhibition of long-term potentiation in rats fed a high-fat diet. Brain Res Bull. 2016 Mar;121:178-85. doi: 10.1016/j.brainresbull.2016.02.005. Epub 2016 Feb 6.

61. Li J, Deng J, Sheng W, Zuo Z. Metformin attenuates Alzheimer's disease-like neuropathology in obese, leptin-resistant mice.PharmacolBiochemBehav. 2012 Jun;101(4):564-74. doi: 10.1016/j.pbb.2012.03.002. Epub 2012 Mar 9.

62. Gupta A, Bisht B, Dey CS. Peripheral insulin-sensitizer drug metformin ameliorates neuronal insulin resistance and Alzheimer's-like

changes. Neuropharmacology. 2011 May;60(6):910-20. doi:

10.1016/j.neuropharm.2011.01.033. Epub 2011 Jan 26.

63. Chen Y, Zhou K, Wang R, Liu Y, Kwak YD, Ma T, Thompson RC, Zhao
Y, Smith L, Gasparini L, Luo Z, Xu H, Liao FF. Antidiabetic
drug metformin (GlucophageR) increases biogenesis of Alzheimer's amyloid
peptides via up-regulating BACE1 transcription.ProcNatlAcadSci U S A. 2009
Mar 10;106(10):3907-12. doi: 10.1073/pnas.0807991106. Epub 2009 Feb 23.

64. Moore EM, Mander AG, Ames D, Kotowicz MA, Carne RP, Brodaty
H, Woodward M, Boundy K, Ellis KA, Bush AI, Faux NG, Martins R, Szoeke
C, Rowe C, Watters DA; AIBL Investigators. . Increased risk of cognitive
impairment in patients with diabetes is associated with metformin.
Diabetes Care. 2013 Oct;36(10):2981-7. doi: 10.2337/dc13-0229. Epub 2013
Sep 5.

65. Imfeld P, Bodmer M, Jick SS, Meier CR. Metformin, other antidiabetic drugs,
and risk of Alzheimer's disease: a population-based case-control study.J Am
Geriatr Soc. 2012 May;60(5):916-21. doi: 10.1111/j.1532-5415.2012.03916.x.
Epub 2012 Mar 28.

66. Hsu CC, Wahlqvist ML, Lee MS, Tsai HN. Incidence of dementia is increased
in type 2 diabetes and reduced by the use of sulfonylureas and metformin.J
Alzheimers Dis. 2011;24(3):485-93. doi: 10.3233/JAD-2011-101524.

67. José A. Luchsinger, Yong Ma, Costas A. Christophi, Hermes Florez, Sherita
H. Golden, Helen Hazuda, JillCrandall, Elizabeth Venditti, Karol Watson, Sus
an Jeffries, Jennifer J. Manly and F. Xavier Pi-Sunyer. Metformin, Lifestyle
Intervention, and Cognition in the Diabetes Prevention Program Outcomes
Study. Diabetes Care 2017 May; dc162376. https://doi.org/10.2337/dc16-2376

68. Orkaby AR, Cho K, Cormack J, Gagnon DR, Driver JA. Metformin vs
    sulfonylurea use and risk of dementia in US veterans aged ≥65 years with
    diabetes.Neurology. 2017 Oct 31;89(18):1877-1885. doi:
    10.1212/WNL.0000000000004586. Epub 2017 Sep 27.

69. Moore E, Mander A, Ames D, Carne R, Sanders K, Watters D. Cognitive
    impairment and vitamin B12: a review. IntPsychogeriatr. 2012 Apr;24(4):541-
    56. doi: 10.1017/S1041610211002511. Epub 2012 Jan 6.

70. Beulens JW, Hart HE, Kuijs R, Kooijman-Buiting AM, Rutten GE. Influence
    of duration and dose of metformin on cobalamin deficiency in type
    2 diabetes patients using metformin. ActaDiabetol. 2015 Feb;52(1):47-53. doi:
    10.1007/s00592-014-0597-8. Epub 2014 Jun 8.

71. Rodríguez-Gutiérrez R, Montes-Villarreal J, Rodríguez-Velver KV, González-
    Velázquez C, Salcido-Montenegro A, Elizondo-Plazas A, González-González
    JG . Metformin Use and Vitamin B12 Deficiency: Untangling the Association.
    Am J Med Sci. 2017 Aug;354(2):165-171. doi: 10.1016/j.amjms.2017.04.010.
    Epub 2017 Jul 8.

72. Kancherla V, Elliott JL Jr, Patel BB, Holland NW, Johnson TM
    2nd, Khakharia A, Phillips LS, Oakley GP Jr, Vaughan CP. Long-
    term Metformin Therapy and Monitoring for Vitamin B12 Deficiency Among
    Older Veterans. J Am Geriatr Soc. 2017 May;65(5):1061-1066. doi:
    10.1111/jgs.14761. Epub 2017 Feb 9.

73. Khattar D, Khaliq F, Vaney N, Madhu SV. Is Metformin-Induced Vitamin
    B12 Deficiency Responsible for Cognitive Decline in Type 2 Diabetes?.
    Indian J Psychol Med. 2016 Jul-Aug;38(4):285-90. doi: 10.4103/0253-
    7176.185952.

74. Biemans E, Hart HE, Rutten GE, Cuellar Renteria VG, Kooijman-Buiting AM, Beulens JW.Cobalamin status and its relation with depression, cognition and neuropathy in patients with type 2 diabetes mellitus using metformin.ActaDiabetol. 2015 Apr;52(2):383-93. doi: 10.1007/s00592-014-0661-4. Epub 2014 Oct 15

75. Parry-Strong A, Langdana F, Haeusler S, Weatherall M, Krebs J. Sublingual vitamin B12 compared to intramuscular injection in patients with type 2 diabetestreated with metformin: a randomised trial. N Z Med J. 2016 Jun 10;129(1436):67-75.

76. Ahmed MA. Metformin and Vitamin B12 Deficiency: Where Do We Stand?. J Pharm Pharm Sci. 2016 Jul - Sep;19(3):382-398. doi: 10.18433/J3PK7P.

77. Svačina Š.[The microbial flora in the digestive tract and diabetes].VnitrLek. 2015 Apr;61(4):361-4.

78. Halmos T, Suba I.[Physiological patterns of intestinal microbiota. The role of dysbacteriosis in obesity, insulin resistance, diabetes and metabolic syndrome].Orv Hetil. 2016 Jan 3;157(1):13-22. doi: 10.1556/650.2015.30296.

79. Alam Q, ZubairAlam M, Karim S, Gan SH, Kamal MA, Jiman-Fatani A, Damanhouri GA, Abuzenadah AM, Chaudhary AG, Haque A. A nanotechnological approach to the management of Alzheimer disease and type 2 diabetes.CNS NeurolDisord Drug Targets. 2014 Apr;13(3):478-86.

80. Sohrab SS, Karim S, Kamal MA, Abuzenadah AM, Chaudhary AG, Al-Qahtani MH, Mirza Z. Bacteriophage--a common divergent therapeutic

approach for Alzheimer's disease and type II diabetes mellitus. CNS
NeurolDisord Drug Targets. 2014 Apr;13(3):491-500.

81. Hirose M, Künstner A, Schilf P, Sünderhauf A, Rupp J, Jöhren
    O, Schwaninger M, Sina C, Baines JF, Ibrahim SM. Mitochondrial gene
    polymorphism is associated with gut microbial communities in mice. Sci
    Rep. 2017 Nov 10;7(1):15293. doi: 10.1038/s41598-017-15377-7.

82. Kelly JR, Minuto C, Cryan JF, Clarke G, Dinan TG. Cross Talk:
    The Microbiota and Neurodevelopmental Disorders. Front Neurosci. 2017 Sep
    15;11:490. doi: 10.3389/fnins.2017.00490. eCollection 2017.

83. Jang SE, Lim SM, Jeong JJ, Jang HM, Lee HJ, Han MJ, Kim DH.
    Gastrointestinal inflammation by gut microbiota disturbance induces memory
    impairment in mice. Mucosal Immunol. 2017 Jun 14. doi:
    10.1038/mi.2017.49. [Epub ahead of print]

84. El Aidy S, Dinan TG, Cryan JF. Gut Microbiota: The Conductor in the
    Orchestra of Immune-Neuroendocrine Communication. ClinTher. 2015 May
    1;37(5):954-67. doi: 10.1016/j.clinthera.2015.03.002. Epub 2015 Apr 3.

85. Jašarević E, Howerton CL, Howard CD, Bale TL. Alterations in the Vaginal
    Microbiome by Maternal Stress Are Associated With Metabolic
    Reprogramming of the Offspring Gut and Brain.Endocrinology. 2015
    Sep;156(9):3265-76. doi: 10.1210/en.2015-1177. Epub 2015 Jun 16.

86. Di Mauro A, Neu J, Riezzo G, Raimondi F, Martinelli D, Francavilla R, Indrio
    F. Gastrointestinal function development and microbiota. Ital J Pediatr. 2013
    Feb 24;39:15. doi: 10.1186/1824-7288-39-15.

87. Martín-Villa JM. Neuroendocrine stimulation of mucosal immune cells in
    inflammatory bowel disease.Curr Pharm Des. 2014;20(29):4766-73

88. Sudo N. Microbiome, HPA axis and production of endocrine hormones in the gut. AdvExp Med Biol. 2014;817:177-94. doi: 10.1007/978-1-4939-0897-4_8.

89. Schroeder BO, Bäckhed F. Signals from the gut microbiota to distant organs in physiology and disease. Nat Med. 2016 Oct 6;22(10):1079-1089. doi: 10.1038/nm.4185. [Epub ahead of print]

90. Alam MZ, Alam Q, Kamal MA, Abuzenadah AM, Haque A. A possible link of gut microbiota alteration in type 2 diabetes and Alzheimer's diseasepathogenicity: an update.CNS NeurolDisord Drug Targets. 2014 Apr;13(3):383-90.

91. Bekkering P, Jafri I, van Overveld FJ, Rijkers GT. The intricate association between gut microbiota and development of type 1, type 2 and type 3diabetes.Expert Rev ClinImmunol. 2013 Nov;9(11):1031-41. doi: 10.1586/1744666X.2013.848793. Epub 2013 Oct 21.

92. . Rotella CM, Monami M, Mannucci E. 2006. Metformin beyond diabetes: new life for an old drug. Curr. Diabetes Rev. 2:307–315. 10.2174/157339906777950651

93. Hardie DG, Ross FA, Hawley SA. 2012. AMPK: a nutrient and energy sensor that maintains energy homeostasis. Nat. Rev. Mol. Cell Biol. 13:251–262. 10.1038/nrm3311

94. Viollet B, Guigas B, Leclerc J, Hebrard S, Lantier L, Mounier R, Andreelli F, Foretz M. 2009. AMP-activated protein kinase in the regulation of hepatic energy metabolism: from physiology to therapeutic perspectives. Acta Physiol. 196:81–98. 10.1111/j.1748-1716.2009.01970.x

95. Foretz M, Hebrard S, Leclerc J, Zarrinpashneh E, Soty M, Mithieux G, Sakamoto K, Andreelli F, Viollet B. 2010. Metformin inhibits hepatic

gluconeogenesis in mice independently of the LKB1/AMPK pathway via a decrease in hepatic energy state. J. Clin. Invest. 120:2355–2369. 10.1172/JCI40671

96. Lee H, Ko G. Effect of Metformin on Metabolic Improvement and Gut Microbiota. Appl Environ Microbiol. 2014 Oct;80(19):5935-43. doi: 10.1128/AEM.01357-14. Epub 2014 Jul 18.

97. Zhang X, Zhao Y, Xu J, Xue Z, Zhang M, Pang X, Zhang X, Zhao L. Modulation of gut microbiota by berberine and metformin during the treatment of high-fat diet-induced obesity in rats. Sci Rep. 2015 Sep 23;5:14405. doi: 10.1038/srep14405.

98. Vijay-Kumar M, Aitken JD, Carvalho FA, Cullender TC, Mwangi S, Srinivasan S, Sitaraman SV, Knight R, Ley RE, Gewirtz AT. Metabolic syndrome and altered gut microbiota in mice lacking Toll-like receptor 5. Science. 2010 Apr 9;328(5975):228-31. doi: 10.1126/science.1179721. Epub 2010 Mar 4

99. Cabreiro F, Au C, Leung KY, Vergara-Irigaray N, Cochemé HM, Noori T, Weinkove D, Schuster E, Greene ND, Gems D. Metformin retards aging in C. elegans by altering microbial folate and methion ine metabolism. Cell. 2013 Mar 28;153(1):228-39. doi: 10.1016/j.cell.2013.02.035.

100.   Lenaerts I., Walker G.A., Van Hoorebeke L., Gems D., Vanfleteren J.R. Dietary restriction of Caenorhabditiselegans by axenic culture reflects nutritional requirement for constituents provided by metabolically active microbes. J. Gerontol. A Biol. Sci. Med. Sci. 2008;63:242–252.

101.   Disentangling type 2 diabetes and metformin treatment signatures in

the human gut microbiota. Forslund K, Hildebrand F, Nielsen T, Falony G, Le

Chatelier E, Sunagawa S, Prifti E, Vieira-Silva S, Gudmundsdottir

V, Pedersen HK, Arumugam M, Kristiansen K, Voigt AY, Vestergaard

H, Hercog R, Costea PI, Kultima JR, Li J, Jørgensen T, Levenez F, Dore

J; MetaHIT consortium, Nielsen HB, Brunak S, Raes J, Hansen T, Wang

J, Ehrlich SD, Bork P, Pedersen O. Nature. 2015 Dec 10;528(7581):262-266.

doi: 10.1038/nature15766. Epub 2015 Dec 2.

102.   Napolitano A, Miller S, Nicholls AW, Baker D, Van Horn S, Thomas

E, Rajpal D, Spivak A, Brown JR, Nunez DJ. Novel Gut-Based Pharmacology

of Metformin in Patients with Type 2 Diabetes Mellitus. PLoS One. 2014

Jul 2;9(7):e100778. doi: 10.1371/journal.pone.0100778. eCollection 2014.

103.   Burton JH, Johnson M, Johnson J, Hsia DS, Greenway FL,

HeimanMLAddition of a Gastrointestinal Microbiome Modulator to

Metformin Improves Metformin Tolerance and Fasting Glucose Levels. J

Diabetes Sci Technol. 2015 Jul; 9(4): 808–814.

104.   Tucker GT, Casey C, Phillips PJ, Connor H, Ward JD, Woods HF.

Metformin kinetics in healthy subjects and in patients with diabetes

mellitus. Br J ClinPharmacol. 1981;12:235–246. doi: 10.1111/j.1365-

2125.1981.tb01206.x

105.   Migoya EM, Bergeron R, Miller JL, et al. Dipeptidyl peptidase-4

inhibitors administered in combination with metformin result in an additive

increase in the plasma concentration of active GLP-

1. ClinPharmacolTher. 2010;88:801–808. doi: 10.1038/clpt.2010.184.

106.   Yee SW, Lin L, Merski M, et al. Prediction and validation of enzyme and transporter off-targets for metformin. J PharmacokinetPharmacodyn. 2015;42:463–475. doi: 10.1007/s10928-015-9436-y.

107.   McCreight LJ, Bailey CJ, Pearson ER. Metformin and the gastrointestinal tract.Diabetologia. 2016; 59: 426–435. doi: 10.1007/s00125-015-3844-9

108.   Wang JH, Bose S, Lim SK, Ansari A, Chin YW, Choi HS, Kim H. Houttuynia cordata Facilitates Metformin on Ameliorating Insulin Resistance Associated with GutMicrobiota Alteration in OLETF Rats. Genes (Basel). 2017 Sep 22;8(10). pii: E239. doi: 10.3390/genes8100239.

109.   Davari S, Talaei SA, Alaei H, Salami M. Probiotics treatment improves diabetes-induced impairment of synaptic activity and cognitivefunction: behavioral and electrophysiological proofs for microbiome-gut-brain axis.Neuroscience. 2013 Jun 14;240:287-96. doi: 10.1016/j.neuroscience.2013.02.055. Epub 2013 Mar 7.

110.   Jack CR, et al. Hypothetical model of dynamic biomarkers of the Alzheimer's pathological cascade. Lancet Neurol. 2010;9:119–128. doi: 10.1016/S1474-4422(09)70299-6.

111.   Pistollato F, et al. Role of gut microbiota and nutrients in amyloid formation and pathogenesis of Alzheimer disease. Nutr. Rev. 2016;74:624–634. doi: 10.1093/nutrit/nuw023.

112.   Gareau MG, Sherman PM, Walker WA. Probiotics and the gut microbiota in intestinal health and disease. Nat. Rev. Gastroenterol. Hepatol. 2010;7:503–514. doi: 10.1038/nrgastro.2010.117.

113.	Savilahti E. Probiotics in the Treatment and Prevention of Allergies in Children. Biosci. Microflora. 2011;30:119–128. doi: 10.12938/bifidus.30.119.

114.	Kafshdooz T, et al. Role of Probiotics in Managing of Helicobacter Pylori Infection: A Review. Drug Res. (Stuttg). 2016;67:88–93. doi: 10.1055/s-0042-116441.

115.	Kondo S, et al. Antiobesity effects of *Bifidobacteriumbreve* strain B-3 supplementation in a mouse model with high-fat diet-induced obesity. Biosci. Biotechnol. Biochem. 2010;74:1656–61. doi: 10.1271/bbb.100267.

116.	Sivan A, et al. Commensal *Bifidobacterium* promotes antitumor immunity and facilitates anti-PD-L1 efficacy. Science. 2015;350:1084–9. doi: 10.1126/science.aac4255

117.	Matsumoto M, Kurihara S, Kibe R, Ashida H, Benno Y. Longevity in mice is promoted by probiotic-induced suppression of colonic senescence dependent on upregulation of gut bacterial polyamine production. PLoS One. 2011;6:e23652. doi: 10.1371/journal.pone.0023652.

118.	Kobayashi Y, Sugahara H, Shimada K, Mitsuyama E, Kuhara T, Yasuoka A, Kondo T, Abe K, Xiao JZ. Therapeutic potential of Bifidobacteriumbreve strain A1 for preventing cognitive impairment in Alzheimer's disease.Sci Rep. 2017 Oct 18;7(1):13510. doi: 10.1038/s41598-017-13368-2.

119.	Liu YW, et al. Psychotropic effects of *Lactobacillus plantarum* PS128 in early life-stressed and naïve adult mice. Brain Res. 2016;1631:1–12. doi: 10.1016/j.brainres.2015.11.018.

120.   Distrutti E, et al. Modulation of intestinal microbiota by the probiotic VSL#3 resets brain gene expression and ameliorates the age-related deficit in LTP. PLoS One. 2014;9:e106503. doi: 10.1371/journal.pone.0106503.

121.   Akbari E, et al. Effect of probiotic supplementation on cognitive function and metabolic status in Alzheimer's Disease: a randomized, double-blind and controlled trial. Front. Aging Neurosci. 2016;8:256. doi: 10.3389/fnagi.2016.00256.

122.   Ait-Belgnaoui A, et al. Probiotic gut effect prevents the chronic psychological stress-induced brain activity abnormality in mice. Neurogastroenterol. Motil. 2014;26:510–20. doi: 10.1111/nmo.12295.[

123.   Takeda S, et al. Validation of Aβ1–40 administration into mouse cerebroventricles as an animal model for Alzheimer disease. Brain Res. 2009;1280:137–147. doi: 10.1016/j.brainres.2009.05.035.

124.   Fung TC, Olson CA, Hsiao EY. Interactions between the microbiota, immune and nervous systems in health and disease. Nat. Neurosci. 2017;20:145–155. doi: 10.1038/nn.4476.

125.   Bravo JA, et al. Ingestion of *Lactobacillus* strain regulates emotional behavior and central GABA receptor expression in a mouse via the vagus nerve. Proc. Natl. Acad. Sci. 2011;108:16050–16055. doi: 10.1073/pnas.1102999108.

126.   Koopman FA, et al. Vagus nerve stimulation inhibits cytokine production and attenuates disease severity in rheumatoid arthritis. Proc. Natl. Acad. Sci. 2016;113:8284–8289. doi: 10.1073/pnas.1605635113.

127.   Schaeffer EL, Figueiro M, Gattaz WF. Insights into Alzheimer disease pathogenesis from studies in transgenic animal models. Clinics. 2011;66:45–54. doi: 10.1590/S1807-59322011001300006

128.   Saito T, et al. Single App knock-in mouse models of Alzheimer's disease. Nat. Neurosci. 2014;17:661–663. doi: 10.1038/nn.3697.

129.   Noble EE, Hsu TM, Kanoski SE. Gut to Brain Dysbiosis: Mechanisms Linking Western Diet Consumption, the Microbiome, and Cognitive Impairment.Front BehavNeurosci. 2017 Jan 30;11:9. doi: 10.3389/fnbeh.2017.00009. eCollection 2017.

130.   Shaik MM, Ahmad S, Gan SH, Abuzenadah AM, Ahmad E, Tabrez S, Ahmed F, Kamal MA. How do periodontal infections affect the onset and progression of Alzheimer's disease?. CNS NeurolDisord Drug Targets. 2014 Apr;13(3):460-6.

131.   ANDREWS P, BORODY T. Bacteriotherapy for chroniconstipation--a long term follow up. Gastroenterology1995; 108: A563.

132.   GOUGH E, SHAIKH H, MANGES AR. Systematic review of intestinal microbiota transplantation (Fecal Bacteriotherapy) for recurrent Clostridium difficile infection. Clin Infect Dis 2011; 53: 994-1002.

YOUR KNOWLEDGE HAS VALUE

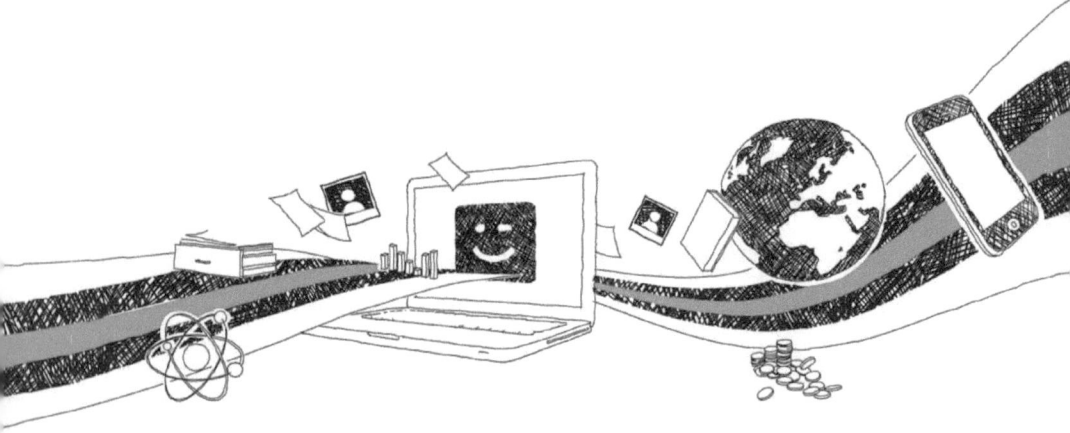

- We will publish your bachelor's and
  master's thesis, essays and papers

- Your own eBook and book -
  sold worldwide in all relevant shops

- Earn money with each sale

Upload your text at www.GRIN.com
and publish for free

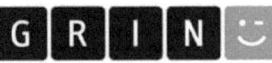